YOUR KNOWLEDGE HAS VALUE

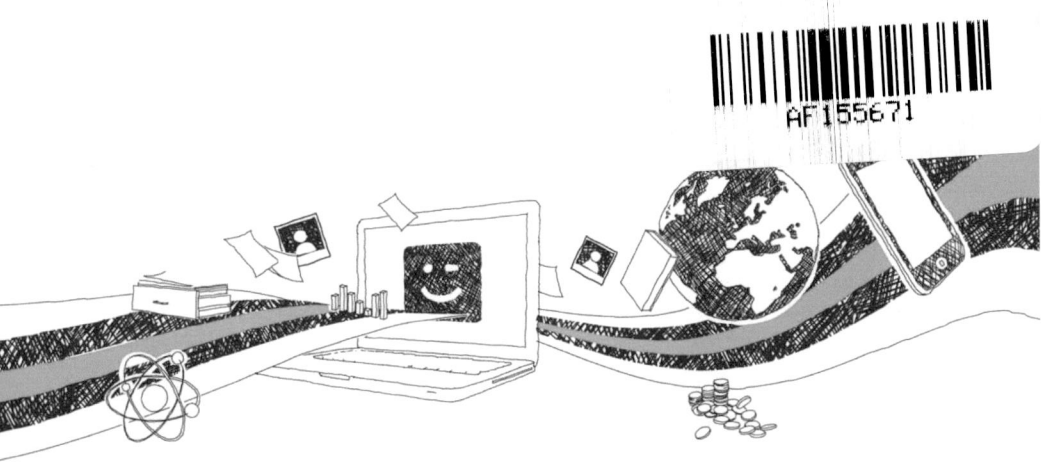
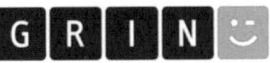

Bibliographic information published by the German National Library:

The German National Library lists this publication in the National Bibliography; detailed bibliographic data are available on the Internet at http://dnb.dnb.de .

Imprint:

Copyright © 2016 GRIN Verlag, Open Publishing GmbH
Print and binding: Books on Demand GmbH, Norderstedt Germany
ISBN: 9783668495395

This book at GRIN:

http://www.grin.com/en/e-book/371249/knowledge-among-mothers-regarding-weaning-practices

Aaqib javed, Ammara Ishtiaq, Khaliq Ur-Rehman, Somia Khan

Knowledge among mothers regarding weaning practices

Cross-sectional descriptive study at the Pediatric Outpatient department of Bahawal Victoria Hospital in Bahawalpur

GRIN Publishing

Title

Knowledge among mothers regarding weaning practices, visiting Pediatric Outpatient department Bahawal Victoria Hospital Bahawalpur.

Authors

1. Dr.Aaqib javed

MBBS, FCPS 1 (Medicine).

Medical officer BHU Adam Wahin,Lodhran.

2. Dr. Ammara Ishtiaq

MBBS, FCPS 1 (Gynae & Obs.).

Women Medical Officer Shahida Islam Hospital Lodhran.

3. Dr. Khaliq-Ur-Rehman

MBBS, FCPS 1 (Medicine).

Medical officer DHQ, Lodhran.

4.Dr. Somia Khan

MBBS, FCPS 1 (Gynae & Obs).

Women Medical officer THQ Taunsa Sharif.

ABSTRACT

Introduction:

Weaning defined as addition of foods in the infant's diet other than mother's milk and slowly Lessing mother's milk. WHO recommends and emphasize on breast feeding for the first four to six months for full term healthy child by a healthy mother. Weaning started after that. WHO and UNICEF also emphasis to continue breast feeding up to the two years of a child's age.

OBJECTIVE:

To evaluate the knowledge awareness and practices of lactating mothers of infants regarding weaning

Study DESIGN:

This cross-sectional descriptive study was conducted at pediatric OPD of BV Hospital Bahawalpur from February 2016 to April 2016.The non - probability convenience sampling method was used to get data from 75 lactating mothers attending outpatient department with their infants.

Data Analysis:

Data was analyzed by SPSS 21 and all results were shown in the form of tables, frequencies and percentages.

RESULTS:

In the present study, 70% of mothers were 20 to 29 years of age, all were housewives, 30% were educated at 10th grade, and 75% lived in the combined family system, mean weaning age was 4-6 month, were more than 65% of sample size. In the interviewed women, 48% used home-made weaning diet. 34% use mixed homemade and commercially refined diets, while 18% use only commercially prepared diets. Breastfeeding was sustained during and after weaning, with 68% of respondents as well as weaning diets.

CONCLUSIONS:

Mothers must be educated about the importance and effectiveness of weaning, age at which weaning starts and the types of weaning diets. This can be achieved through the use of LHWs, LHVs and by use of media. The importance of continued breastfeeding after weaning should be emphasized.

Key Words:

Mothers; Practices; Infants: Weaning.

Content

Introduction 4

Results 6

Discussion...10

Conclusions 12

References 13

INTRODUCTION

Weaning defined as addition of foods in the infant's diet other than mother's milk and slowly Lessing mother's milk.[1] WHO recommends and emphasize on breast feeding for the first four to six months for full term healthy child by a healthy mother. Weaning started after that.[2] WHO and UNICEF also emphasis to continue breast feeding up to the age of two years of a child.[3] It is observed that all importance put on weaning age without added physiological, psychological economic and nutritional benefits of early weaning.[4] Severe health complications can occur in infants due to delayed weaning as after six month of age alone mother's milk is not sufficient to fulfill the nutritional requirement of the child. Mother's milk contains insufficient quantity of zinc, iron and vitamin A for the nursing baby.

Delayed weaning causes Protein energy malnutrition due to which severe Neurological manifestation can occur.[5] In underdeveloped countries bottle feeding is used as alternate of mother's milk that also have its own disadvantages like diarrhea, gastritis, allergic conditions and dental caries. Infant mortality rate is about 4.5 times higher in children using bottle feed as compared to breast feeding Childs.[6] Breast feeding reduces 30% risk of breast cancer (pre-menopausal).[7]

Factors that affecting weaning vary according to socioeconomic condition of the population like education, culture, norms and believes and taboos. They also vary according to regional distribution of the world. In united state avg. weaning age was from 2.5 to 3 years the common reason for starting of weaning was said to be "child-led" and that was accomplished slowly. Comprehensive nursing was infrequent. In Kuwait, They use artificial feeding immediately after birth. The breast feeding rate was 26% while bottle feeding rate was 42%.Between 3 months to 5 months of ages, fruit juices, cereal products like biscuits and cerelac given to the child.[8]

Working mothers and the mothers having handsome income status weaning early as compared to housewives and the mothers having poor socio economic status. The most frequent used weaning diet was adult diet like ingera, kitta, and bread followed by egg. In Pakistan according to NATIONAL NUTRITION SURVEY 68% children used other diet than milk between the ages of seven to nine months of age; 30-50% infants not received semi solid or solid food even at the age of one to two years of age. Start of solid diet was also late even in rural areas of Pakistan.[9]

Weaning food prepared in underdeveloped countries in unhygienic conditions by using contaminated water that cause weaning diarrhea in Childs. This causes dilemma to mother and child; to wean or not wean which termed as "Weanling dilemma", so these questions still alive when to start weaning, how to wean and what to wean. The purpose of this study was to access mean weaning age, types of weaning foods, continuation of mother's milk and source of information for weaning practices.

OBJECTIVE:

To evaluate the knowledge awareness and practices of lactating mothers of infants regarding weaning

Methodology and material:

This cross-sectional descriptive study was conducted at pediatric OPD of BV Hospital Bahawalpur from February 2016 to April 2016.The non - probability convenience sampling method was used to get data from 75 lactating mothers attending outpatient department with their infants. A structured Questionnaire used to collect data from mothers. Data was entered and analyzed using SPSS software version 21. Descriptive statistical determination is in the form of percentages, frequencies and tables.

Results

The Socio demographic profile of 75 mothers presented in Table 1

Most of the Mothers 51 (68%) were age group 20-29 years of age, while 18 (24%) were in 30-39 years age group.33 (44%) were illiterate , 14 (18%) were primary pass ,23(30%) were metric and 2(4%) were intermediate or above.

54(72%) women were having one to two child while 7(9%) had five to six Childs. 39(52%) had monthly income 3000-5000 rupees while 11 (14%) had earning less than three thousand rupee per month, 7(10%) had monthly income above ten thousand rupee.

Occupational status of fathers revealed that 30(40%) fathers were working on daily wages basis, 21 (28%) were having their own business, 19(26%) were regular in employment and 5 (6%) did not specify their earning sources. 56 (75%) were living in combined family system. When inquired about the age of youngest child 27 (35%) had younger Childs within the age group of 23 to 24 months and 36 (47%) mothers were having children less than one 12 months of age. From Youngest children 49(65%) were males and 26(35%) were females.

34(46%) infants had adding up of solid food in diet at the age of 5 to 6 months, 22 (30%) had weaning diet the age of 6 moths,12(16%) started weaning food at the age of 3 to 4 months of age and 3 (4%) started solid food at 1-2 months of age. Four children (5%) were not started weaning yet.

Thirty six percent mothers started weaning by her selves, 33% started weaning as advised by doctor, and 15% started weaning because of thinking of low breast milk, 11 mothers started weaning as counseled by LHVs or inspired by media.[Figure-1]

Food items given at weaning with percentage of infants given in Table 2.Breast feeding along with weaning continued by 51(68%) and was discontinued by 21 (27%).

Table No.1

Socio-Demographic profile	No of Mothers	Percentage
Age in years		
20-29	51	68%
30-39	18	24%
40-49	6	8%
Education		
illiterate	33	44%
Primary	14	18%
middle	3	4%
metric	23	30%
Intermediate or above	2	4%
Number of Children		
1-2	54	72%
3-4	14	19%
5-6	7	9%
Monthly Family income(Rupees)		
< 3000	11	14%
3000-5000	39	52%
6000-10000	18	24%
>10000	7	10%

Socio-Demographic Profile of 75 Mothers

Table No.2

Food items given at weaning

FOOD	No of Mothers	Percentage
Bread	18	24%
Chappati	28	38%
Rice	50	66%
Legumes	9	12%
Eggs	30	40%
Milk	39	52%
Meat	9	12%
Fish	4	5%
Chicken	11	15%
Fruit	26	35%
Vegetables	15	20%
Butter	2	2%
Oils	4	5%
Ghee	4	5%
Honey	11	15%

Figure -1

Reason for weaning at a particular age

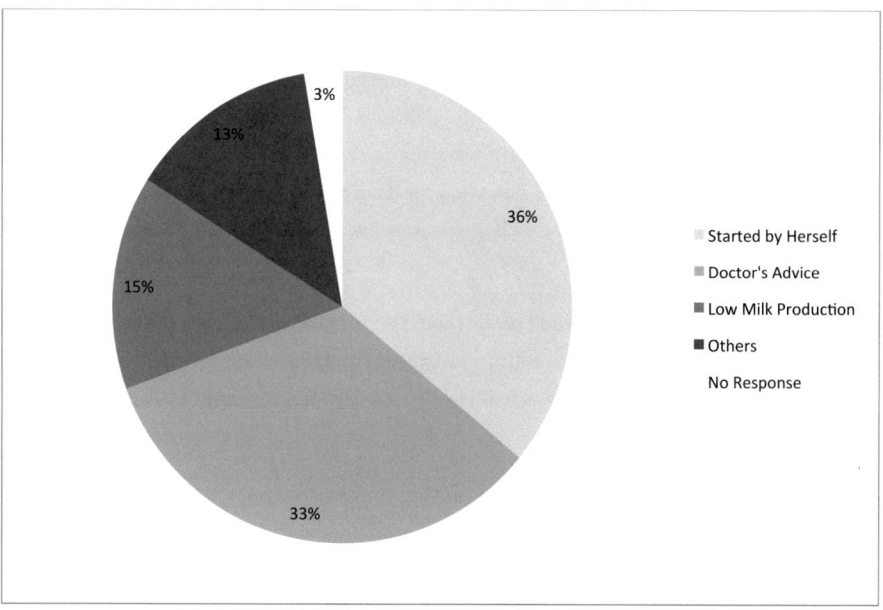

Discussion

Feeding practices are important determinants of future physical and mental well-being of Childs. The practice of weaning low in nutrient density and high bulk infant formulas for weaning is a well known problem all over the world. Early introduction of solid diets and unsanitary practices in infants prone to malnutrition, stunting, infection and high mortality.[10] In Pakistan according to NATIONAL NUTRITION SURVEY 68% children used other diet than milk between the ages of seven to nine months of age; 30-50% infants not received semi solid or solid food even at the age of one to two years of age. The mean weaning age is 8 months in Baluchistan.[11] The incidence and duration of breastfeeding reduced while bottles and solid foods are introduced earlier.[12]

The first part of our study focused on the mean age of weaning and socio demographic factors that could influence weaning potential. This study showed that the mean age of weaning was between 4 and 6 months, which was based on WHO criteria and suggested weaning exercises.

This finding with the results of the study was carried out in weaning practices, a low socioeconomic group.[13] For weaning, the onset period in mostly (30% of the highest percentage) for more than 6 months, and it was further observed in this study that the majority of mothers 68% were between the ages of 20-29 years old. No one is under 19 years of age and less than 9% is older than 40 years of age. All mothers were interviewed, most were not well educated, 66% less than matriculation, and 30% of mothers were metric pass.

A similar study conducted in Kuwait the fact that the educational status was lower about 72% of mothers was illiterate or under metric and its associated mothers were often delayed in weaning to children until the 6 months or more. The study also showed that for all interviewed housewives, 66% of respondents' husbands earning was Rs 5000 per month or less. Among them, 11 had incomes lower than Rs. 3000. Studies conducted in Ethiopia have interfered that mothers having better economic status had 2 times better chances of starting early weaning as compared to mothers from poor background. A similar co relation was seen in mothers those who were working women with the onset of weaning age in their children. Mothers working outside of their homes had 3.3 time better chances to start early weaning. In our study 75% lived in the combined family system. It is related to another finding in our study 60% of mothers were having six or more than six family members living with them. 54(72%) women were having one to two child while 7(9%) had five to six Childs, and 47% of mothers having children below one year of age.

Our research focuses on another part of the weaning practice. It is interesting to note that about 36% of mothers start giving their children a semi-solid food based on their own mother's sensation and instinct.[14] Jalil et al reported that 50% of the urban poor began to be weaned because of insufficient supply of milk. The finding was supported by another study in the United States where the youngest child was weaned for 63.5% of the reasons for the exploration. Weaning is said to be child led. In the present study, 33% of mothers consulted physicians for weaning. This finding is contrary to the fact that 55% of women in Glasgow-based research revealed that they received formal information about weaning from health visitor.[15] In this study rice was given the highest priority as a weaning diet (66%), followed by milk (52%), eggs (40%), chappati (38%) and fruits (35%). In addition, ghee and butter turned out to be the most unpopular baby weaning food. Cultural differences in weaning practices are observed all over the world, although low - income groups use starchy foods more than high - protein diets. In Africa, the most popular weaning foods were cooked bananas (96%), followed by cow milk, corn porridge, millet porridge and potatoes as weaning diet. These findings also supported by a study on aboriginal infants and children.[16] Another study conducted in West Africa showed that people with low socioeconomic classes rarely eat meat, eggs or fish for their infant's diet; not only because of socioeconomic factors, but that social taboos and ignorance added factors.[17] In the interviewed women, 48% used home-made weaning diet. 34% use mixed homemade and commercially refined diets, while 18% use only commercially prepared diets. This is similar in Kuwait, revealing that 63.5% of mothers introduced homemade weaned foods, although only 19% relied on commercial preparations.[18]

Regardless of age at onset of weaning, Breast feeding along with weaning continued by 51(68%) and was discontinued by 21 (27%).Elsewhere studies have shown that bottle feeding is not just used to give milk, but they are also used to give semi-solid cereals as well. Therefore, bottle feeding is now socially and culturally accepted by the Pakistani guidelines.[19]

Conclusions

It is suggest that mothers need to be educated about the importance of weaning, weaning age and the type of infant weaning diets. This can be achieved through the use of LHV and LHW and the mass media. It suggested that the nutrition education program should be reactivated to promote breastfeeding and weaning mother's practices. The procedure should be directed to all mothers, especially in their first infants and working mothers. It should focus on promoting breastfeeding not only after delivery but also on prolonging its duration for two years. The period prescribed by the World Health Organization should be emphasized, along with its advantages and disadvantages early and delayed weaning adhering to our benefits.

References

1. World Health Organization (WHO). Complementary Feeding: Family Foods for Breast-feeding Children. Geneva, 2000.
2. Kikafunda JK. Walker AF and JK Tumwine. Weaning Foods and Practices in Central Uganda: A Cross-sectional Study. African Journal of Food, Agriculture, Nutrition and Development. 2003; 3(2).
3. Ahmad Z. Kyi DW and Isa AR. Breast-feeding and Weaning Practices in Rural Communities of Kelantan.MaI J Nutr2. 1996; 148-154.
4. Aregai WG. Determinants of Weaning Practices. EJHD. 2000:14(2): 183-189.
5. Odebode TO and Odebode SO. Protein Energy Malnutrition and the Nervous System: the Impact of Sochio-economic Condition, Weaning Practice, Infection and Food Intake, an Experience in Nigeria. PJN. 2005; 4 (5): 304-309.
6. Sharnim S, Jamalvi SW and Naz F. Determinants of Bottle Use amongst Economically DisadvantagedMothers. JAMC. 2006; 18(1).
7. Sugarman M, Kendall-Tackett KA. Weaning Ages in a Sample of American Women Who Practice Extended Breastfeeding. 1995; 34(12): 642-647.
8. Fawzia A., Al-Awadi and Ezzat KA. Recent Trends in Infant Feeding Patterns and Weaning in Kuwait. EMHJ .1997; 3(3):501 -510.
9. Khaleel M, Rashid J, Khan MMN and Zaheer A. Assessment of Knowledge and Practice Regarding Weaning Among Mothers of Infants 4-12 Months of Age in a Semi-Urban Population. JPPA. 1-5.
10. UNICEF and Nutritional cell Punjab. Pakistan. Training of health care providers in mother and child nutrition. Revised edition 1995.
11. Government of Pakistan. National Nutrition survey. Nutrition Division, National Institute of Health,Islamabad. 1998.
12. Ahmad Z, Kyi DW and Isa AR. Breast feeding and weaning practices in rural communities of Kelantan.MaI J Nutr 2.1996; 148-54.
13. Shamin S. weaning practices in pen-urban low socioeconomic groups; JCPSP.2005 Mar; 15(3): 129-32.
14. Jalil F, Karlberg J, Hanson LA and Lindbald BS. Growth disturbances in an urban area of Lahore, Pakistan related to feeding patterns, infectios and age, sex,socio economic factors and reasons. Acta Paediatr.1989; 350(2S):14-54.
15. Shirley SA, Reilly J, Edwards C and Durnin J. Weaning practice in Glasgow longitudinal infant growth study;Arch Dis Child. 1998 August; 79:153-156.
16. Gracey M. Infant feeding and weaning practices in an urbanizing traditional, hunter-gatherer society.Pediatrics.2000; 106(5): 1276-1277.
17. Onofiok N and Nnanyelugo DO. Nutrient intake of infants of high and low socio-economic group in Nsukka, Nigeria. Occasional paper. Department of home sciences and nutrition. University of Nigeria, Nsukkal 992.

18. Shamim S, Jamalvi W, Naz F. Determinants of bottle use amongst economically disadvantaged mothers. JAMC. 2006; 18(1): 1-3.
19. Osama NA and El Subhan FF. Infant feeding practices in Al Ain — United Arab Emirates. Eastern Med Health J. 1992; 2:1003-10.

YOUR KNOWLEDGE HAS VALUE

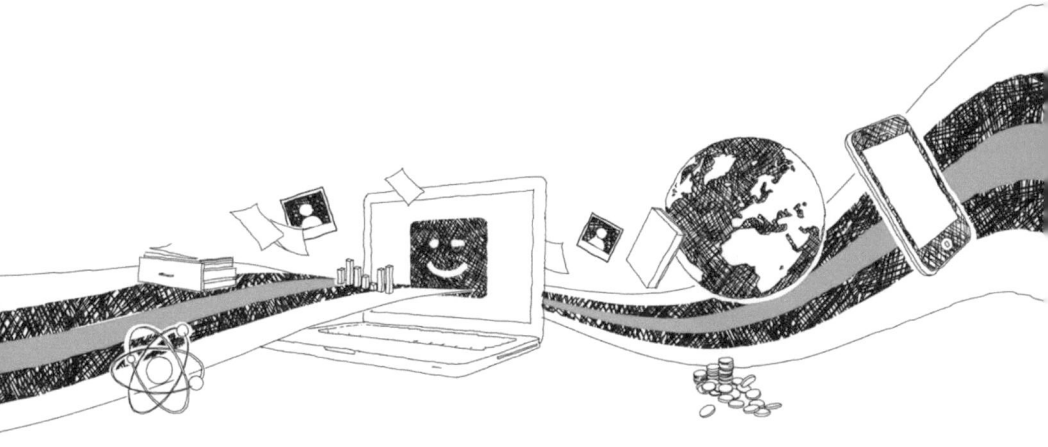

- We will publish your bachelor's and master's thesis, essays and papers

- Your own eBook and book - sold worldwide in all relevant shops

- Earn money with each sale

Upload your text at www.GRIN.com and publish for free

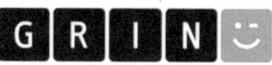